# CSID

# DIET

## COOKBOOK

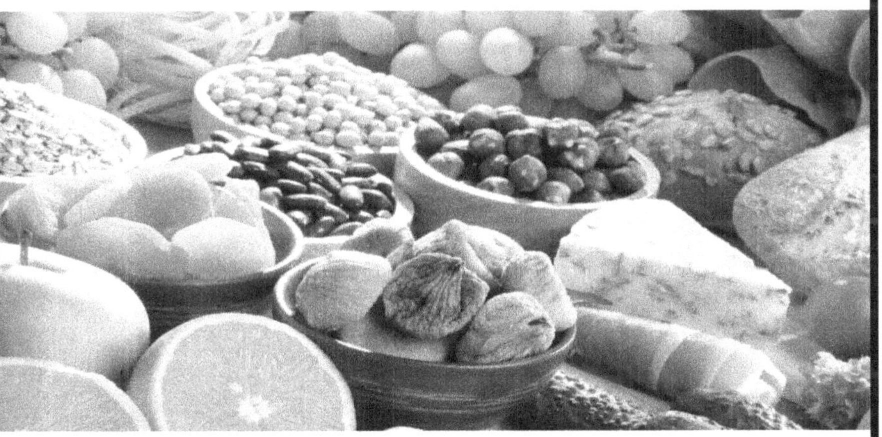

**Low-Sucrose, Low-Starch Recipes for Thriving with Sucrase-Isomaltase Deficiency and Reclaiming Your Health in 2024!"**

Avery Stoneheart

# CONTENTS

# INTRODUCTION

My name is **Avery Stoneheart**, and I am a **doctor and diet instructor** with over 20 years of experience guiding people on their dietary journeys. I have dedicated my life to helping individuals achieve their health goals and lead a more fulfilling life through proper nutrition and diet.

Throughout my career, I have witnessed countless success stories from people who have transformed their lives by making simple changes to their diet. One such story is that of **Alexandra**, a mother of two who struggled with **chronic digestive issues and fatigue for years.** After following the CSID diet and incorporating the recipes in this book, she not only saw a significant improvement in her **symptoms but also experienced increased energy and overall well-being.**

In this cookbook, I have compiled a collection of delicious and nutritious recipes that cater to those with **Congenital Sucrase-Isomaltase Deficiency (CSID)** and those looking to improve their overall health.

Each recipe has been carefully crafted to provide a balance of essential nutrients and to be easy to prepare, ensuring that you can enjoy a variety of tasty and satisfying meals without compromising your health.

As you start this trip in the kitchen, keep in mind that even small changes can have a big effect on your health. I'm sure that the foods and health tips in this book will help you make healthy changes in your life and reach your health goals.

Wishing you the best of health,
*Avery Stoneheart, PhD Diet Instructor*

# CHAPTER ONE

## What is CSID?

CSID, or Congenital Sucrase-Isomaltase Deficiency, is a rare genetic condition that affects the body's ability to digest certain sugars and starches. People with CSID are born with a deficiency in the sucrase-isomaltase enzyme, which is responsible for breaking down sucrose (table sugar) and isomaltase (a type of starch). As a result, undigested sugars and starches remain in the digestive system, causing a range of uncomfortable and painful symptoms.

*Some of the symptoms that people with CSID may experience include the following:*

- Diarrhea
- Abdominal pain
- Bloating, and excessive gas.
- Malnutrition.

These symptoms can vary in severity and may appear shortly after birth or develop later in life. In infants, CSID can lead to failure to thrive, while in older children and adults, it can cause chronic digestive issues and nutrient deficiencies.

The diagnosis of CSID typically involves a combination of medical history, physical examination, and laboratory tests. A hydrogen breath test can be used to measure the amount of undigested sugars in the breath after consuming a test meal. A small intestine biopsy may also be performed to measure sucrase-isomaltase enzyme activity.

There is no cure for CSID, but it can be effectively managed through dietary changes. A CSID diet involves avoiding or limiting foods that are high in sucrose and starch, such as table sugar, fruits, grains, and starchy vegetables. Instead, individuals with CSID should focus on consuming foods that are low in sucrose and starch, such as lean proteins, vegetables, and healthy fats.

In some cases, a medication called Sucraid may be prescribed to help manage CSID symptoms. Sucraid is an artificial sucrase enzyme that can be taken before meals to aid in the digestion of sucrose.

**In conclusion**, CSID is a rare genetic condition that affects the body's ability to digest certain sugars and starches. By understanding the symptoms, diagnosis, and management options, individuals with CSID can make informed decisions about their diet and lifestyle to minimize discomfort and maintain optimal health.

# The Importance of a CSID-Friendly Diet

A CSID-friendly diet is essential for individuals with **Congenital Sucrase-Isomaltase Deficiency (CSID),** a rare genetic condition that affects the body's ability to digest certain sugars and starches. This diet can help alleviate uncomfortable and painful digestive symptoms, promote overall health, and improve quality of life.

In this book, we'll explore the **benefits of a CSID-friendly diet and provide you with a collection of delicious and nutritious recipes to support your dietary needs.**

1. **Relief from digestive symptoms:** A CSID-friendly diet is specifically designed to avoid or limit foods that contain sucrose and starch, which can be difficult for individuals with CSID to digest. By following this diet, you can experience significant relief from common digestive symptoms such as diarrhea, bloating, gas, and abdominal pain.

2. **Nutrient absorption:** When undigested sugars and starches remain in the digestive system, they can interfere with the absorption of essential nutrients. A CSID-friendly diet helps to prevent this issue, ensuring that your body can effectively absorb the nutrients it needs for optimal health.

3. **Healthy weight maintenance:** A CSID-friendly diet encourages the consumption of whole, unprocessed foods that are rich in essential nutrients. This can help you maintain a healthy weight and reduce the risk of obesity and other related health issues.

4. **Improved quality of life:** By alleviating uncomfortable digestive symptoms and promoting overall health, a CSID-friendly diet can significantly improve your quality of life. You'll feel better, have more energy, and be able to enjoy a wider variety of foods without worrying about triggering digestive discomfort.

In this cookbook, you'll find a **wealth of delicious and easy-to-prepare recipes** that cater to the needs of individuals with CSID. From breakfast to dinner and everything in between, our recipes are designed to provide you with the nutrition you need while also being enjoyable to eat.

Use our cookbook as a springboard to explore a world of CSID-friendly recipes that are full of flavor, healthy, and easy to whip up. Embrace a healthier, happier you while bidding farewell to gastrointestinal distress.

# HOW THIS COOKBOOK CAN HELP

Our cookbook is designed to help individuals with Congenital Sucrase-Isomaltase Deficiency (CSID) and those looking to improve their overall health by providing a collection of delicious and nutritious recipes that cater to a CSID-friendly diet.

***Here's how this book can help you on your dietary journey:***

1. **Easy-to-follow recipes:** Our cookbook features a wide range of recipes that are easy to prepare, making it simple for you to incorporate a CSID-friendly diet into your daily routine.

2. **Nutritional guidance:** Each recipe in this book is carefully crafted to provide a balance of essential nutrients, ensuring that you get the nourishment your body needs while following a CSID-friendly diet.

3. **Variety of options:** From breakfast to dinner and everything in between, our cookbook offers a diverse selection of recipes to suit every taste and preference.

This variety helps to keep your diet interesting and enjoyable, making it easier to stick to a CSID-friendly diet in the long term.

4. **Tips and advice:** Throughout the book, we provide helpful tips and advice on how to manage a CSID-friendly diet, making it easier for you to navigate the challenges of this dietary restriction and maintain a healthy lifestyle.

5. **Success stories:** Our cookbook includes real-life success stories from individuals who have improved their health and well-being by following a CSID-friendly diet. These stories can serve as inspiration and motivation as you embark on your own dietary journey.

6. **FAQ:** We have also included a frequently asked questions section in the book, addressing common concerns and providing answers to help you better understand and navigate the CSID-friendly diet.

This section aims to provide clarity and alleviate any doubts or uncertainties you may have about the dietary restrictions and guidelines.

By following the recipes and tips in this book, you'll be well on your way to enjoying the benefits of a CSID-friendly diet, such as better health, fewer stomach problems, and better absorption of nutrients. Accept the power of a CSID-friendly diet and begin your path to wellness and happiness.

# CHAPTER TWO

## BREAKFAST RECIPES

*Savory Scrambled Eggs with Avocado:*

**Ingredients:**

- 2 eggs

- 1 tablespoon butter or extra virgin olive oil

- 1/4 avocado, diced

- 1/4 cup alfalfa sprouts

- Salt and pepper to taste

**Cooking Time: 10 minutes**

**Instructions:**

1. Melt butter or oil in a small skillet over medium heat.

2. Add eggs and scramble until cooked through.

3. Stir in avocado, alfalfa sprouts, salt, and pepper.

4. Serve immediately.

## Nutritional Facts (per serving)

- Calories: 300
- Protein: 18g
- Fat: 20g
- Carbohydrates: 10g
- Fiber: 5g

## Tips:

- Use pasture-raised eggs for an extra boost of nutrients.
- Add chopped vegetables, such as spinach, mushrooms, or bell peppers, to increase fiber and vitamins.
- Serve with a side of whole-grain toast or avocado for a balanced meal.

## *Protein-Packed Frittata:*

### Ingredients:

- 1 tablespoon butter or extra virgin olive oil
- 1/2 cup broccoli florets
- 1/2 cup zucchini, diced
- 1/4 cup cooked chicken, shredded
- 1/4 cup cheddar cheese, shredded
- 3 eggs
- Salt and pepper to taste

### Cooking Time: 20 minutes

### Instructions:

1. Preheat oven to 350 degrees F (175 degrees C).
2. Melt butter or oil in a small oven-safe skillet over medium heat.
3. Add broccoli and zucchini and cook until softened.
4. Stir in cooked chicken, cheddar cheese, eggs, salt, and pepper.
5. Transfer skillet to oven and bake for 15-20 minutes, or until frittata is set.
6. Cut into wedges and serve.

## Nutritional Facts (per serving)

- Calories: 350
- Protein: 25g
- Fat: 25g
- Carbohydrates: 15g
- Fiber: 5g

## Tips:

- Use a variety of vegetables to increase the nutrient content of your frittata.
- Add lean protein sources, such as chopped chicken or turkey, for an extra boost of protein.
- Sprinkle with fresh herbs, such as basil or parsley, for added flavor.

## *Creamy Spinach and Artichoke Dip with Veggies:*

## Ingredients:

- 1 tablespoon butter or extra virgin olive oil
- 1/2 cup artichoke hearts, chopped
- 1/2 cup frozen spinach, thawed and drained
- 1/4 cup ricotta cheese
- 1/4 cup plain yogurt
- 1/4 cup grated Parmesan cheese
- Salt and pepper to taste

## Preparation Time: 15 minutes

## Instructions:

1. Melt butter or oil in a small saucepan over medium heat.
2. Add artichoke hearts and cook until softened.
3. Stir in spinach, ricotta cheese, yogurt, Parmesan cheese, salt, and pepper.
4. Serve warm with your favorite vegetables for dipping.

## Nutritional Facts (per serving)

- Calories: 250
- Protein: 10g
- Fat: 20g
- Carbohydrates: 10g
- Fiber: 5g

## Tips:

- Use low-fat Greek yogurt instead of sour cream to reduce the fat content.
- Add chopped vegetables, such as carrots, celery, or cucumbers, for extra crunch and nutrients.
- Serve with whole-grain crackers or vegetable sticks for a healthier option.

## *Citrus Berry Salad*

### Ingredients:

- Mixed greens: Spinach, baby arugula, romaine, or a combination
- Citrus fruits: Oranges, grapefruits, mandarins, clementines, blood oranges (any combination you like)
- Berries: Strawberries, blueberries, raspberries, blackberries (any combination you like)
- Other fruits: Sliced grapes, kiwi, mango, pineapple (optional)
- Nuts or seeds: Chopped almonds, walnuts, pecans, sunflower seeds, pumpkin seeds (optional)
- Cheese: Feta, goat cheese, ricotta salata (optional)
- Dressing: Vinaigrette, honey-lime dressing, poppyseed dressing (recipe below)

### Preparation Time: 10 minutes

## Instructions:

1. Wash and dry the greens.
2. Peel and segment the citrus fruits, removing any membranes.
3. Hull and slice the strawberries, and rinse the other berries.
4. Prepare any other fruits you are using, such as slicing grapes or chopping mango.
5. Toast the nuts or seeds in a dry pan over medium heat, if using.
1. To make a simple vinaigrette dressing, whisk together olive oil, lemon juice or vinegar, Dijon mustard, a pinch of sugar, and salt and pepper to taste, vinegar, Dijon mustard, sugar, salt, and pepper]
6. In a large bowl, combine the greens, citrus fruits, berries, other fruits (if using), nuts or seeds (if using), and cheese (if using).
7. Drizzle with the dressing and toss gently to coat.

## Nutritional Facts (per serving)

- Calories: 150
- Protein: 2g
- Fat: 5g
- Carbohydrates: 25g
- Fiber: 5g

## Tips:

- For a sweeter salad, use more berries and less citrus.
- For a tart and tangy salad, use more grapefruit and less sweet oranges.
- Add grilled chicken or shrimp for a heartier salad.
- Get creative with the dressing! Try a balsamic vinaigrette, a honey-lime dressing, or a poppyseed dressing.
- Top the salad with fresh herbs like mint or basil.
- Use a variety of citrus fruits, such as oranges, grapefruit, and tangerines, for a burst of flavor and vitamin C.
- Add mixed berries, such as strawberries, blueberries, and raspberries, for additional antioxidants and fiber.
- Toss with a light vinaigrette or drizzle with honey for a touch of sweetness.

## Refreshing Fruit Salad with Yogurt:

## Ingredients:

- 1 cup mixed berries
- 1 cup chopped papaya
- 1/2 cup blueberries
- 1/4 cup plain yogurt
- 1 tablespoon honey
- 1 teaspoon lemon juice

## Preparation Time: 10 minutes

## Instructions:

1. Combine all ingredients in a medium bowl.

2. Chill for at least 30 minutes before serving.

## Nutritional Facts (per serving)

- Calories: 200
- Protein: 10g
- Fat: 5g
- Carbohydrates: 30g
- Fiber: 5g

## Tips:

- Use a variety of fruits, such as melons, pineapple, and mango, for a tropical twist.
- Add chopped nuts and seeds for extra crunch and protein.
- Top with a dollop of Greek yogurt for added creaminess and protein.

## Nutrient-Rich Smoothie:

### Ingredients:

- 1 cup unsweetened almond milk
- 1/2 cup frozen raspberries
- 1/2 banana
- 1/4 cup plain yogurt
- 1 tablespoon honey
- 1 teaspoon vanilla extract

### Preparation Time: 5 minutes

### Instructions:

1. Combine all ingredients in a blender and blend until smooth.
2. Enjoy immediately.

### Nutritional Facts (per serving)

- Calories: 300
- Protein: 15g
- Fat: 10g
- Carbohydrates: 40g
- Fiber: 5g

## Tips:

- Use frozen fruits for a thicker consistency and extra nutrients.

- Add a scoop of protein powder for an extra boost of protein.

- Blend in a handful of spinach or kale for added vitamins and minerals.

## *Flavorful Avocado Toast with Eggs:*

### Ingredients:

- 1 slice whole-grain toast
- 1/4 avocado, mashed
- 2 eggs, fried or poached
- Salt and pepper to taste

### Preparation Time: 10 minutes

### Instructions:

1. Toast bread until lightly browned.
2. Spread avocado on toast.
3. Top with fried or poached eggs.
4. Season with salt and pepper to taste.

### Nutritional Facts (per serving)

- Calories: 300
- Protein: 15g
- Fat: 20g
- Carbohydrates: 20g
- Fiber: 5g

### Tips:

- Use whole-grain bread for a healthier option.
- Mash avocado with a fork and spread it evenly on the bread.
- Top with poached or fried eggs for added protein.
- Season with salt, pepper, and other herbs and spices to taste.

## Energizing Trail Mix:

### Ingredients:

- 1/2 cup Brazil nuts

- 1/4 cup unsweetened shredded coconut

- 1/4 cup pine nuts

- 1/4 cup sesame seeds

- 1 tablespoon honey

### Preparation Time: 5 minutes

### Instructions:

1. Combine all ingredients in a medium bowl.

2. Store in an airtight container at room temperature.

### Nutritional Facts (per serving)

- Calories: 200

- Protein: 10g

- Fat: 15g

- Carbohydrates: 15g

- Fiber: 5g

## Tips:

- Combine a variety of nuts and seeds, such as almonds, cashews, sunflower seeds, and pumpkin seeds, for a balanced mix of healthy fats, protein, and fiber.

- Add dried fruits, such as raisins, cranberries, and apricots, for a burst of sweetness and extra antioxidants.

- Spice up your trail mix with a pinch of cinnamon, nutmeg, or ginger for a warm and cozy flavor.

- Store your trail mix in an airtight container in the refrigerator for up to two weeks.

## Decadent Chocolate Avocado Mousse:

### Ingredients:

- 1 ripe avocado
- 1/4 cup unsweetened cocoa powder
- 1/4 cup plain yogurt
- 1 tablespoon honey
- 1 teaspoon vanilla extract

### Preparation Time: 10 minutes

### Instructions:

1. Combine all ingredients in a food processor and blend until smooth.
2. Chill for at least 30 minutes before serving.

### Nutritional Facts (per serving)

- Calories: 250
- Protein: 5g
- Fat: 20g
- Carbohydrates: 20g
- Fiber: 10g

## Tips:

- Use very ripe avocados for a smooth and creamy texture.

- Add a touch of honey or maple syrup for extra sweetness, if desired.

- For a richer chocolate flavor, use dark chocolate or cocoa powder.

- Decorate your mousse with fresh berries, a sprinkle of cocoa powder, or shaved chocolate for a gourmet touch.

# Refreshing Coconut Water Popsicles:

## Ingredients:

- 1 cup pure coconut water

- 1 tablespoon honey

- 1/2 cup mixed berries

- 1 teaspoon lemon juice

Preparation Time: 10 minutes (plus freezing time)

## Instructions:

1. Combine all ingredients in a blender and blend until smooth.

2. Pour mixture into popsicle molds and freeze for at least 4 hours.

## Nutritional Facts (per serving)

- Calories: 60

- Protein: 1g

- Fat: 0g

- Carbohydrates: 15g

- Fiber: 0g

## Tips:

- Use pure coconut water for the best flavor and hydration benefits.
- Add a squeeze of lime juice or a splash of fruit juice for extra flavor and vitamin C.
- For a sweeter treat, blend in some honey or maple syrup.
- Freeze the popsicles for at least 4 hours or overnight before enjoying.

# CHAPTER THREE

## LUNCH RECIPES

*Hearty Beef and Vegetable Stew:*

**Ingredients:**

- 1 tablespoon butter or extra virgin olive oil
- 1 pound beef stew meat, cut into cubes
- 2 cups broccoli florets
- 2 cups carrots, chopped
- 2 cups celery, chopped
- 1 cup beef broth
- Salt and pepper to taste

**Cooking Time: 2 hours**

**Instructions:**

1. Melt butter or oil in a large Dutch oven over medium heat.
2. Add beef stew meat and cook until browned on all sides.
3. Stir in broccoli, carrots, celery, and beef broth.
4. Bring to a boil, then reduce heat and simmer for 1-2 hours, or until beef is tender.

5.  Season with salt and pepper to taste.

6.  Serve over mashed potatoes or rice.

## Nutritional Facts (per serving)

-   Calories: 400

-   Protein: 30g

-   Fat: 20g

-   Carbohydrates: 30g

-   Fiber: 10g

## Tips:

-   Use lean cuts of beef, such as sirloin or chuck roast, to reduce the fat content.

-   Add a variety of vegetables, such as carrots, celery, potatoes, and peas, for increased fiber and nutrient content.

-   Use a low-sodium broth to control sodium intake.

-   Serve with a side of whole-grain bread or brown rice for a complete meal.

## Savory Pork Lettuce Wraps with Avocado Salsa:

### Ingredients:

- 1 tablespoon butter or extra virgin olive oil
- 1 pound ground pork
- 1/2 cup cabbage, shredded
- 1/4 cup green onions, chopped
- 1 tablespoon tahini paste
- 1 tablespoon lemon juice
- 1 teaspoon honey
- 1/2 avocado, diced
- 1/4 cup raspberries
- 12 lettuce leaves

### Preparation Time: 15 minutes

### Instructions:

1. Melt butter or oil in a large skillet over medium heat.
2. Add ground pork and cook until browned.
3. Stir in cabbage, green onions, tahini paste, lemon juice, honey, and salt and pepper to taste.
4. Cook until cabbage is softened.

5. Meanwhile, prepare the avocado salsa by combining diced avocado, raspberries, and salt and pepper to taste.

6. To assemble, fill each lettuce leaf with a scoop of pork mixture and top with avocado salsa.

## Nutritional Facts (per serving)

- Calories: 350
- Protein: 25g
- Fat: 15g
- Carbohydrates: 25g
- Fiber: 5g

## Tips:

- Use lean ground pork or turkey to reduce the fat content.
- Add chopped vegetables, such as bell peppers, onions, and mushrooms, for extra flavor and nutrients.
- Use a light vinaigrette or a dollop of Greek yogurt for a healthier dressing option.
- Serve with a variety of lettuce leaves, such as romaine, butterhead, or bibb lettuce.

# Refreshing Lamb Salad with Lemon Vinaigrette:

## Ingredients:

- 1 tablespoon butter or extra virgin olive oil
- 1 pound lamb chops, grilled and sliced
- 2 cups mixed greens
- 1/2 cup cherry tomatoes, halved
- 1/2 cucumber, sliced
- 1/4 cup plain yogurt
- 1 tablespoon lemon  juice
- 1 teaspoon honey
- Salt and pepper to taste

## Preparation Time: 20 minutes

## Instructions:

1. Grill lamb chops over medium heat until cooked to desired doneness.
2. Slice lamb chops and set aside.
3. Toss mixed greens, cherry tomatoes, and cucumber together in a large bowl.
4. In a small bowl, whisk together yogurt, lemon juice, honey, salt, and pepper.

5.  Drizzle dressing over salad and toss to coat.

6.  Top with sliced lamb and serve.

## Nutritional Facts (per serving)

- Calories: 300

- Protein: 20g

- Fat: 15g

- Carbohydrates: 20g

- Fiber: 5g

## Tips:

- Use lean lamb cuts, such as loin chops or sirloin, to reduce the fat content.

- Add a variety of mixed greens, such as spinach, arugula, and kale, for increased fiber and nutrient content.

- Use a light lemon vinaigrette made with olive oil, lemon juice, Dijon mustard, and herbs for a refreshing flavor.

- Serve with a side of whole-grain crackers or pita bread for a complete meal.

## *Flavorful Fish Tacos with Mango Salsa:*

### Ingredients:

- 1 tablespoon butter or extra virgin olive oil
- 2 cod fillets
- 1/2 cup mango, diced
- 1/4 cup avocado, diced
- 1 tablespoon lime juice
- 1 teaspoon honey
- 12 corn tortillas
- Coleslaw (optional)

### Preparation Time: 20 minutes

### Instructions:

1. Melt butter or oil in a large skillet over medium heat.
2. Add cod fillets and cook until cooked through.
3. Flake cod and set aside.
4. In a medium bowl, combine diced mango, avocado, lime juice, honey, and salt and pepper to taste.
5. Warm corn tortillas in a skillet over medium heat.

6. To assemble, fill each tortilla with flaked cod, mango salsa, and coleslaw, if desired.

## Nutritional Facts (per serving)

- Calories: 350
- Protein: 25g
- Fat: 15g
- Carbohydrates: 30g
- Fiber: 5g

## Tips:

- Use white-fleshed fish, such as cod, tilapia, or halibut, for a lower-fat option.

- Prepare the mango salsa in advance for a fresh and flavorful topping.

- Use corn tortillas or whole-wheat tortillas for a healthier option.

- Add chopped vegetables, such as onions, tomatoes, and cilantro, for extra flavor and nutrients.

## *Citrus Berry Salad*

### Ingredients:

- Mixed greens: Spinach, baby arugula, romaine, or a combination
- Citrus fruits: Oranges, grapefruits, mandarins, clementines, blood oranges (any combination you like)
- Berries: Strawberries, blueberries, raspberries, blackberries (any combination you like)
- Other fruits: Sliced grapes, kiwi, mango, pineapple (optional)
- Nuts or seeds: Chopped almonds, walnuts, pecans, sunflower seeds, pumpkin seeds (optional)
- Cheese: Feta, goat cheese, ricotta salata (optional)
- Dressing: Vinaigrette, honey-lime dressing, poppyseed dressing (recipe below)

### Preparation Time: 10 minutes

## Instructions:

1. Wash and dry the greens.
2. Peel and segment the citrus fruits, removing any membranes.
3. Hull and slice the strawberries, and rinse the other berries.
4. Prepare any other fruits you are using, such as slicing grapes or chopping mango.
5. Toast the nuts or seeds in a dry pan over medium heat, if using.
6. To make a simple vinaigrette dressing, whisk together olive oil, lemon juice or vinegar, Dijon mustard, a pinch of sugar, and salt and pepper to taste, vinegar, Dijon mustard, sugar, salt, and pepper]
7. In a large bowl, combine the greens, citrus fruits, berries, other fruits (if using), nuts or seeds (if using), and cheese (if using).
8. Drizzle with the dressing and toss gently to coat.

## Nutritional Facts (per serving)

- Calories: 150
- Protein: 2g
- Fat: 5g
- Carbohydrates: 25g
- Fiber: 5g

## Tips:

- For a sweeter salad, use more berries and less citrus.
- For a tart and tangy salad, use more grapefruit and less sweet oranges.
- Add grilled chicken or shrimp for a heartier salad.
- Get creative with the dressing! Try a balsamic vinaigrette, a honey-lime dressing, or a poppyseed dressing.
- Top the salad with fresh herbs like mint or basil.
- Use a variety of citrus fruits, such as oranges, grapefruit, and tangerines, for a burst of flavor and vitamin C.
- Add mixed berries, such as strawberries, blueberries, and raspberries, for additional antioxidants and fiber.
- Toss with a light vinaigrette or drizzle with honey for a touch of sweetness.

# Seared Salmon with Roasted Brussels Sprouts and Lemon-Dill Sauce

## Ingredients:

### For the salmon:

- 2 salmon fillets (6 ounces each)
- 1 tablespoon olive oil
- 1/2 teaspoon dried thyme
- 1/4 teaspoon salt
- 1/4 teaspoon black pepper

### For the roasted Brussels sprouts:

- 1 pound Brussels sprouts, trimmed and halved
- 1 tablespoon olive oil
- 1/2 tcaspoon salt
- 1/4 teaspoon black pepper

### For the lemon-dill sauce:

- 1/4 cup plain Greek yogurt
- 1/4 cup chopped fresh dill
- 1 tablespoon lemon juice
- 1/4 teaspoon salt
- 1/4 teaspoon black pepper

## Instructions:

1. Preheat oven to 400°F (200°C).

2. For the salmon: In a small bowl, whisk together olive oil, thyme, salt, and pepper. Brush both sides of the salmon fillets with the mixture.

3. Heat a large skillet over medium-high heat. Add the salmon fillets, skin-side down, and cook for 3-4 minutes, or until the skin is crispy.

## Salmon fillets searing in a skillet

4. Flip the salmon fillets and cook for an additional 2-3 minutes, or until cooked through.

5. For the roasted Brussels sprouts: Toss the Brussels sprouts with olive oil, salt, and pepper. Spread on a baking sheet in a single layer.

## Brussels sprouts tossed with olive oil, salt, and pepper

6. Roast for 20-25 minutes, or until tender and browned.

7. For the lemon-dill sauce: In a small bowl, whisk together Greek yogurt, dill, lemon juice, salt, and pepper.

8.  To serve, plate the salmon fillets and top with roasted Brussels sprouts. Spoon the lemon-dill sauce over the top.

## Nutritional Facts (per serving)

- Calories: 450
- Protein: 35g
- Fat: 25g
- Carbohydrates: 30g
- Fiber: 10g

## Cooking Time: 30 minutes

## Tips:

- Use skin-on salmon fillets for added omega-3 fatty acids.
- Roast Brussels sprouts with olive oil, salt, and pepper for a healthy and flavorful side dish.
- Make a light lemon-dill sauce using Greek yogurt, lemon juice, dill, and a pinch of sweetener.

# Nutrient-Rich Turkey Burgers with Zucchini Fries:

## Ingredients:

- 1 pound ground turkey
- 1/4 cup chopped onion
- 1/4 cup chopped bell pepper
- 1 tablespoon tahini paste
- 1 tablespoon lemon juice
- 1 teaspoon honey
- 2 zucchinis, peeled and cut into wedges
- Olive oil
- Salt and pepper to taste

## Cooking Time: 20 minutes

## Instructions:

1. Preheat oven to 400 degrees F (200 degrees C).
2. In a large bowl, combine ground turkey, onion, bell pepper, tahini paste, lemon juice, honey, salt, and pepper.
3. Form mixture into patties.
4. Grill or cook patties in a skillet over medium heat until cooked through.

5. Toss zucchini wedges with olive oil, salt, and pepper.

6. Spread zucchini wedges on a baking sheet and bake for 20-25 minutes, or until tender.

7. Serve turkey burgers with zucchini fries.

## Nutritional Facts (per serving)

- Calories: 350
- Protein: 30g
- Fat: 15g
- Carbohydrates: 25g
- Fiber: 5g

## Tips:

- Use lean ground turkey or a combination of turkey and ground chicken for a lower-fat option.

- Add chopped vegetables, such as carrots, celery, and onions, to the burger patties for extra flavor and nutrients.

- Bake or grill the zucchini fries instead of frying them for a healthier option.

- Serve the burgers on whole-wheat buns or lettuce wraps.

## *Energizing Chicken Salad with Fruit and Nuts:*

### Ingredients:

- 1 pound cooked chicken, shredded
- 1 cup mixed greens
- 1/2 cup grapes, halved
- 1/4 cup strawberries, sliced
- 1/4 cup walnuts, chopped
- 1 tablespoon tahini paste
- 1 tablespoon lemon juice
- 1 teaspoon honey

### Preparation Time: 15 minutes

### Instructions:

1. In a large bowl, combine cooked chicken, mixed greens, grapes, strawberries, walnuts, tahini paste, lemon juice, honey, salt, and pepper.
2. Toss to coat.
3. Serve immediately.

## Nutritional Facts (per serving)

- Calories: 250
- Protein: 20g
- Fat: 10g
- Carbohydrates: 20g
- Fiber: 5g

## Tips:

- Use cooked or canned chicken breast for a quick and easy option.

- Add chopped fruits, such as apples, grapes, and celery, for sweetness and fiber.

- Mix in chopped nuts, such as almonds, pecans, or walnuts, for added protein and healthy fats.

- Serve the chicken salad on whole-wheat bread or crackers.

## *Refreshing Salmon Salad with Fennel and Berries:*

### Ingredients:

- 1 pound cooked salmon, flaked
- 1 cup mixed greens
- 1/2 cup fennel, shaved
- 1/4 cup blueberries
- 1/4 cup raspberries
- 1 tablespoon tahini paste
- 1 tablespoon lemon juice
- 1 teaspoon honey

### Preparation Time: 20 minutes

### Instructions:

1. In a large bowl, combine cooked salmon, mixed greens, fennel, blueberries, raspberries, tahini paste, lemon juice, honey, salt, and pepper.
2. Toss to coat.
3. Serve immediately.

## Nutritional Facts (per serving)

- Calories: 300
- Protein: 25g
- Fat: 15g
- Carbohydrates: 20g
- Fiber: 5g

## Tips:

- Use cooked or canned salmon for a quick and easy option.
- Add finely chopped fennel bulb for a unique flavor and added fiber.
- Mix in fresh berries, such as strawberries, blueberries, and raspberries, for sweetness and antioxidants.
- Serve the salmon salad on whole-grain bread, crackers, or lettuce cups.

## *Flavorful Veggie Burgers with Avocado Spread:*

### Ingredients:

- 1 cup cooked quinoa, cooled
- 1 cup grated carrots
- 1/2 cup chopped zucchini
- 1/4 cup chopped onion
- 1 tablespoon tahini paste
- 1 tablespoon lemon juice
- 1 teaspoon honey
- 1 avocado, mashed
- Salt and pepper to taste

### Cooking Time: 20 minutes

### Instructions:

1. In a large bowl, combine cooked quinoa, grated carrots, chopped zucchini, chopped onion, tahini paste, lemon juice, honey, salt, and pepper.
2. Form mixture into patties.
3. Grill or cook patties in a skillet over medium heat until cooked through.

4.  To assemble, spread avocado mash on buns and top with veggie burgers.

5.  Serve immediately.

## Nutritional Facts (per serving)

- Calories: 300

- Protein: 15g

- Fat: 15g

- Carbohydrates: 30g

- Fiber: 10g

## Tips:

- Use a combination of vegetables, such as carrots, zucchini, bell peppers, and onions, for a flavorful and nutritious burger patty.

- Make a creamy avocado spread by mashing avocado with lemon juice, salt, and pepper.

- Toast whole-wheat buns or use lettuce wraps for a healthier option.

- Top the veggie burgers with your favorite toppings, such as lettuce, tomato, and sprouts.

# CHAPTER FOUR

## DINNER RECIPES

### Pan-Seared Lamb Chops with Roasted Brussels Sprouts and Lemon Tahini Sauce:

**Ingredients:**

- 2 lamb chops, bone-in
- 1 tablespoon butter or extra virgin olive oil
- Salt and pepper to taste
- 1 head Brussels sprouts, trimmed and halved
- 1 tablespoon tahini paste
- 1 tablespoon lemon juice
- 1 teaspoon honey

**Instructions:**

1. Preheat oven to 400 degrees F (200 degrees C).
2. Season lamb chops with salt and pepper.
3. Melt butter or oil in a large skillet over medium-high heat.
4. Sear lamb chops for 2-3 minutes per side, or until browned.

5. Transfer lamb chops to a baking sheet and roast for 5-10 minutes, or until cooked to desired doneness.

6. While lamb chops are cooking, toss Brussels sprouts with olive oil, salt, and pepper.

7. Spread Brussels sprouts on a baking sheet and roast for 15-20 minutes, or until tender.

8. To make the sauce, whisk together tahini paste, lemon juice, honey, and salt and pepper to taste.

9. Serve lamb chops with roasted Brussels sprouts and lemon tahini sauce.

## *Creamy Salmon Pasta with Lemon and Herbs:*

### Ingredients:

- 1 pound salmon fillets, cut into 1-inch pieces
- 1 tablespoon butter or extra virgin olive oil
- 1/2 cup chopped onion
- 1/4 cup chopped bell pepper
- 1 tablespoon chopped fresh parsley
- 1 tablespoon chopped fresh dill
- 1 teaspoon lemon zest
- 1/4 cup plain yogurt
- 1/4 cup grated Parmesan cheese
- 1/4 cup chopped fresh basil
- 1 pound pasta, cooked according to package directions

### Instructions:

1. Melt butter or oil in a large skillet over medium heat.
2. Add onion and bell pepper and cook until softened.
3. Stir in parsley, dill, lemon zest, yogurt, Parmesan cheese, and basil.
4. Add cooked salmon and heat through.
5. Toss cooked pasta with the salmon sauce.
6. Serve immediately.

# Hearty Beef Stew with Vegetables and Herbs:

## Ingredients:

- 1 tablespoon butter or extra virgin olive oil
- 1 pound beef stew meat, cut into cubes
- 2 cups broccoli florets
- 2 cups carrots, chopped
- 2 cups celery, chopped
- 1 cup beef broth
- 1 tablespoon Worcestershire sauce
- 1 teaspoon dried thyme
- 1 teaspoon dried oregano
- Salt and pepper to taste

## Instructions:

1. Melt butter or oil in a large Dutch oven over medium heat.

2. Add beef stew meat and cook until browned on all sides.

3. Stir in broccoli, carrots, celery, beef broth, Worcestershire sauce, thyme, oregano, salt, and pepper.

4. Bring to a boil, then reduce heat and simmer for 1-2 hours, or until beef is tender.

5. Serve over mashed potatoes or rice.

## Flavorful Chicken Stir-Fry with Vegetables and Brown Rice:

### Ingredients:

- 1 tablespoon butter or extra virgin olive oil
- 1 pound boneless, skinless chicken breasts, cut into strips
- 1 cup broccoli florets
- 1 cup sliced bell peppers
- 1/2 cup sliced onion
- 1 tablespoon soy sauce
- 1 tablespoon honey
- 1 teaspoon grated ginger
- 1 teaspoon minced garlic
- 1 cup cooked brown rice

### Instructions:

1. Heat butter or oil in a large skillet or wok over medium-high heat.
2. Add chicken and stir-fry until cooked through.
3. Add broccoli, bell peppers, and onion and stir-fry for 2-3 minutes, or until softened.
4. Stir in soy sauce, honey, ginger, and garlic.
5. Stir-fry for 1 minute more.
6. Serve over cooked brown rice.

## Refreshing Shrimp Salad with Lemon and Herbs:

### Ingredients:

- 1 pound cooked shrimp, peeled and deveined
- 1/2 cup chopped celery
- 1/4 cup chopped onion
- 1/4 cup plain yogurt
- 1 tablespoon lemon juice
- 1 teaspoon honey
- Salt and pepper to taste

### Instructions:

1. Combine cooked shrimp, celery, onion, yogurt, lemon juice, honey, salt, and pepper in a large bowl.
2. Toss to coat.
3. Serve immediately

## Savory Pork Tenderloin with Roasted Apples and Sweet Potatoes

### Ingredients:

- 1 (2-pound) pork tenderloin
- 2 tablespoons olive oil
- 1 teaspoon salt
- 1/2 teaspoon black pepper
- 2 apples, peeled and cored
- 1 sweet potato, peeled and diced

### Instructions:

1. Preheat oven to 400 degrees F (200 degrees C).

2. In a small bowl, combine olive oil, salt, and pepper. Rub the mixture all over the pork tenderloin.

3. Place the pork tenderloin in a roasting pan and roast for 25-30 minutes, or until cooked through.

4. While the pork is roasting, toss the apples and sweet potatoes with olive oil, salt, and pepper.

5. Spread the apples and sweet potatoes around the pork tenderloin and roast for an additional 15-20 minutes, or until the apples are tender and the sweet potatoes are cooked through.

6. Let the pork rest for 10 minutes before slicing.

7. Serve with roasted apples and sweet potatoes.

# Creamy Lemon Chicken with Zucchini and Herbs

## Ingredients:

- 1 pound boneless, skinless chicken breasts, cut into bite-sized pieces
- 1 tablespoon olive oil
- 1/2 cup chopped onion
- 1 zucchini, diced
- 1/2 cup plain yogurt
- 1/4 cup lemon juice
- 1 teaspoon dried oregano
- 1/2 teaspoon salt
- 1/4 teaspoon black pepper
- 1/4 cup chopped fresh basil

## Instructions:

1. Heat olive oil in a large skillet over medium heat.
2. Add chicken and cook until browned on all sides.
3. Add onion and zucchini and cook until softened.
4. In a small bowl, whisk together yogurt, lemon juice, oregano, salt, and pepper.
5. Pour the yogurt mixture over the chicken and vegetables.
6. Bring to a simmer and cook for 5-7 minutes, or until the chicken is cooked through.
7. Stir in basil and serve.

# Hearty Beef Chili with Black Beans and Corn

## Ingredients:

- 1 tablespoon olive oil
- 1 pound ground beef
- 1 onion, chopped
- 2 cloves garlic, minced
- 1 tablespoon chili powder
- 1 teaspoon cumin
- 1 teaspoon smoked paprika
- 1/2 teaspoon salt
- 1/4 teaspoon black pepper
- 1 (14.5-ounce) can diced tomatoes, undrained
- 1 (15-ounce) can black beans, drained and rinsed
- 1 (15-ounce) can corn, drained and rinsed

## Instructions:

1. Heat olive oil in a large pot over medium heat.
2. Add ground beef and cook until browned.
3. Add onion and garlic and cook until softened.
4. Stir in chili powder, cumin, smoked paprika, salt, and pepper.
5. Cook for 1 minute more.
6. Stir in diced tomatoes, black beans, and corn.
7. Bring to a boil, then reduce heat and simmer for 20-30 minutes, or until thickened.
8. Serve with your favorite toppings.

# Flavorful Salmon with Roasted Vegetables

## Ingredients:

- 1 pound salmon fillet
- 1 tablespoon olive oil
- 1 teaspoon dried thyme
- 1/2 teaspoon salt
- 1/4 teaspoon black pepper
- 1 broccoli florets
- 1 carrot, sliced
- 1/2 cup chopped onion

## Instructions:

1. Preheat oven to 400 degrees F (200 degrees C).
2. Rub olive oil, thyme, salt, and pepper all over the salmon fillet.
3. Place the salmon fillet on a baking sheet.
4. Arrange the broccoli florets, carrots, and onions around the salmon.
5. Roast for 15-20 minutes, or until the salmon is cooked through and the vegetables are tender.

## *Shrimp Scampi with Linguine*

### Ingredients:

- 12 ounces gluten-free linguine or fettuccine (such as brown rice or lentil pasta)
- 1 tablespoon olive oil
- 1 tablespoon ghee or unsalted butter
- 2 cloves garlic, minced
- 1/2 teaspoon dried oregano
- 1/4 teaspoon red pepper flakes (optional)
- 1 pound large shrimp, peeled and deveined
- 1/2 cup dry white wine or chicken broth
- 1/4 cup lemon juice
- 1/4 cup chopped fresh parsley
- Salt and pepper to taste

### Instructions:

1. Cook the pasta according to package directions.
2. While the pasta is cooking, heat the olive oil and ghee or butter in a large skillet over medium heat. Add the garlic, oregano, and red pepper flakes (if using) and cook for 30 seconds, or until fragrant.

3. Add the shrimp to the skillet and cook for 2-3 minutes per side, or until pink and cooked through.

4. Pour in the white wine or chicken broth and lemon juice. Bring to a simmer and cook for 1-2 minutes, scraping up any browned bits from the bottom of the pan.

5. Drain the pasta and add it to the skillet with the shrimp and sauce. Toss to coat.

6. Garnish with chopped parsley and serve immediately.

## Nutritional Information:

1. Per serving (based on 4 servings):
2. Calories: 450
3. Fat: 18g
4. Carbohydrates: 45g (net 25g)
5. Fiber: 5g
6. Protein: 35g
7. Sugar: 2g

## Tips:

1. You can use frozen shrimp, thawed, in this recipe.

2. If you don't have white wine or chicken broth, you can use water and add a squeeze of lemon juice for flavor.

3. For a richer flavor, you can add a tablespoon of grated Parmesan cheese to the sauce.

4. Serve this dish with a side of roasted vegetables or a simple salad.

# CHAPTER FIVE

## DRINKS AND JUICES RECIPES

### Refreshing Avocado Smoothie:

**Ingredients:**

1 ripe avocado
1 cup unsweetened almond milk
1/2 cup frozen kiwifruit
1 tablespoon honey

**Instructions:**

- Combine all ingredients in a blender and blend until smooth.
- Enjoy immediately.

### Energizing Raspberry Limeade:

**Ingredients:**

- 1 cup raspberries
- 1 cup unsweetened almond milk
- 1/2 cup lime juice
- 1 tablespoon honey

**Instructions:**

1. Combine all ingredients in a blender and blend until smooth.
2. Strain the mixture through a fine-mesh sieve to remove seeds. Serve chilled.

## Tropical Papaya Smoothie:

### Ingredients:

- 1 cup frozen papaya chunks
- 1 cup unsweetened coconut water
- 1 tablespoon honey

### Instructions:

1. Combine all ingredients in a blender and blend until smooth.
2. Enjoy immediately.


## Antioxidant-Rich Blueberry Blast:

### Ingredients:

- 1 cup blueberries
- 1 cup unsweetened almond milk
- 1 tablespoon honey

### Instructions:

1. Combine all ingredients in a blender and blend until smooth.
2. Enjoy immediately.

## Tart and Tangy Currant Spritzer:

### Ingredients:

- 1 cup currants

- 1 cup unsweetened sparkling water

- 1 tablespoon honey

### Instructions:

1. Muddle currants in a glass using a muddler.

2. Add sparkling water and honey.

3. Stir and serve chilled.


## Zesty Gooseberry Fizz:

### Ingredients:

- 1 cup gooseberries

- 1 cup unsweetened sparkling water

- 1 tablespoon honey

### Instructions:

1. Muddle gooseberries in a glass using a muddler.

2. Add sparkling water and honey.

3. Stir and serve chilled.

## Lemon-Aid Refreshment:

### Ingredients:

- 1 lemon, juiced
- 1 cup unsweetened sparkling water
- 1 tablespoon honey

### Instructions:

1. Combine lemon juice, sparkling water, and honey in a glass.
2. Stir and serve chilled.


## Lime Cooler:

### Ingredients:

- 1 lime, juiced
- 1 cup unsweetened sparkling water
- 1 tablespoon honey

### Instructions:

1. Combine lime juice, sparkling water, and honey in a glass.
2. Stir and serve chilled.

## Avocado-Kiwi Cooler:

### Ingredients:

- 1/2 avocado, diced

- 1 kiwi, peeled and diced

- 1 cup unsweetened almond milk

- 1 tablespoon honey

### Instructions:

- Combine all ingredients in a blender and blend until smooth.
- Enjoy immediately.

## Raspberry-Papaya Delight:

### Ingredients:

- 1/2 cup raspberries
- 1/2 cup frozen papaya chunks
- 1 cup unsweetened almond milk
- 1 tablespoon honey

### Instructions:

1. Combine all ingredients in a blender and blend until smooth.
2. Enjoy immediately.

# CONCLUSION

In conclusion, the CSID diet has been a valuable resource for individuals dealing with congenital sucrose-isomaltase deficiency. By providing a comprehensive guide to managing this condition through dietary modifications, we hope to have empowered our readers to make informed choices about the foods they consume.

The benefits of following a CSID-friendly diet are numerous. Not only does it alleviate the gastrointestinal symptoms associated with CSID, but it also promotes overall health and well-being. By focusing on a variety of nutritious and delicious foods that are low in sucrose and starch, individuals can enjoy a balanced and satisfying diet while managing their condition.

We encourage you to try the recipes provided in this cookbook and share your feedback with us. Your experiences and insights can help us improve and expand our collection of CSID-friendly recipes in future editions.

As you continue your journey with the CSID diet, we encourage you to explore more CSID-friendly options and adapt the diet to your individual needs. Remember, everyone's experience with CSID is unique, and it may take some trial and error to find the right balance for you.

We hope that this cookbook has provided you with the tools and information necessary to manage your CSID and enjoy a fulfilling and healthy diet. Thank you for joining us on this journey, and we look forward to hearing about your experiences with the CSID diet.

# BONUS SECTION

## CSID-Friendly Grocery List

This grocery list will guide you through essential ingredients for creating delicious and nutritious meals following the CSID guidelines.

### Protein:

**Meats and poultry:** Choose lean cuts of beef, pork, lamb, fish, turkey, or chicken.

**Cooking Tips:** Avoid breaded meats and opt for cooking methods like grilling, baking, roasting, or pan-frying with healthy oils like extra virgin olive oil, avocado oil, or canola oil. Season with salt and pepper as desired.

Eggs are a versatile source of protein, perfect for breakfast, lunch, or dinner. Consider hard-boiled, scrambled, or omelets.

### Vegetables:

**Cruciferous:** broccoli, cabbage, kale, turnips, and Brussels sprouts—rich in vitamins and fiber. Steam, roast, or stir-fry lightly.

**Leafy Greens:** spinach, arugula, mustard greens, and romaine lettuce are excellent sources of vitamins and minerals. Enjoy in salads, wraps, or smoothies.

**Other Choices:** Green beans, zucchini, radishes, and artichoke hearts add variety and flavor to your diet. Try grilling, roasting, or using in stir-fries or soups.

## Fruits:

**Low-Fructose:** Avocado, kiwifruit, raspberries, papaya, blueberries, currants, gooseberries, lemon, and lime provide vitamins, minerals, and antioxidants without triggering CSID symptoms. Enjoy it fresh, in smoothies, or as baked goods.

## Dairy:

**Plain Varieties:** unsweetened milk, ricotta cheese, plain cottage cheese, sour cream, butter, whipping cream, and hard cheeses like cheddar, Colby, mozzarella, Swiss, Parmesan, and provolone—good sources of calcium and protein. Choose lactose-free options if needed.

**Nuts and seeds:**

**Limited Quantities:** Brazil nuts, unsweetened coconut, pine nuts, sesame seeds, and tahini paste provide healthy fats and minerals. Enjoy them in moderation, as they can contain some starch.

## Sweeteners:

**CSID-Safe Options:** Acesulfame-K, aspartame, glucose, honey (use sparingly), maltitol, and sorbitol. Choose alternatives to sucrose (table sugar) and fructose.

## Additional Tips:

- Focus on whole, unprocessed foods whenever possible.
- Check ingredient labels carefully for hidden sugars and starches.
- Don't hesitate to modify recipes to suit your needs and preferences.

# FAQs about the CSID Diet:

## Basics:

1. **What is CSID?** CSID (Congenital Sucrase-Isomaltase Deficiency) is a rare genetic disorder where the body lacks enzymes to digest certain sugars, mainly sucrose and starch.

2. **What are the symptoms of CSID?** Common symptoms include bloating, gas, diarrhea, abdominal pain, and malnutrition.

3. **How is CSID diagnosed?** Diagnosis typically involves a combination of genetic testing, small bowel biopsy, and hydrogen breath tests.

4. **Is there a cure for CSID?** There is no cure, but dietary management can effectively control symptoms and improve overall health.

## Diet:

5. **What is the goal of the CSID diet?** The goal is to limit or avoid foods containing sucrose and starch while ensuring adequate nutrition.

6.  **What foods are restricted on the CSID diet?** Foods high in sucrose (table sugar) and starchy carbs are generally restricted, including most fruits, grains, and processed foods.

7.  **Can I eat vegetables on the CSID diet?** Most vegetables are low in sucrose and starch and are safe to eat, with some exceptions like corn and peas.

8.  **Can I eat rice with CSID?** White rice is high in starch and not recommended, but some rice alternatives like brown rice or wild rice may be tolerated in small amounts.

9.  **Can I drink milk with CSID?** Lactase-free milk is usually safe, as lactose doesn't contain sucrose.

10. **What are some alternative sweeteners safe for CSID?** Stevia, monk fruit extract, and xylitol are some safe options in moderation.

## Food Choices:

11. **What fruits have no sucrose?** Berries like strawberries, raspberries, and blueberries are low in sucrose.

12. **What are 3 foods that contain sucrose?** Table sugar, fruits like bananas, and processed foods like cookies and cakes are high in sucrose.

13. **Which fruits are high in sucrose?** Fruits like grapes, mangoes, pineapples, and bananas have higher sucrose content.

14. **What are some good protein sources for the CSID diet?** Meat, poultry, fish, eggs, tofu, and legumes are excellent protein sources.

15. **Can I eat gluten-free on the CSID diet?** While gluten and sucrose are different, a gluten-free diet can help simplify meal planning, as many processed gluten-free options are also high in sucrose.

## Living with CSID:

16. **Can I eat out with CSID?** Planning ahead and choosing restaurants with clear menus can help. Consider bringing your own snacks or asking about modifications.

17. **How can I manage social events on the CSID diet?** Explain your condition politely to hosts and bring your own safe snacks or dishes to share.

18. **Are there support groups for people with CSID?** Online and local support groups can offer valuable information, tips, and emotional support.

19. **Can I travel with CSID?** Planning meals and snacks in advance, researching local grocery stores and restaurants, and informing airlines about your needs can help make travel smoother.

20. **Is there research on potential treatments for CSID?** Research into enzyme replacement therapy and gene therapy options is

ongoing, offering hope for future advancements in managing CSID.